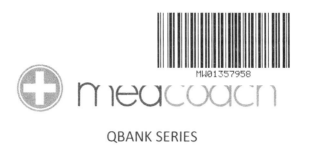

QBANK SERIES

ACING THE PREVIEW EXAM

MedCoach 2023

Table of Contents

Introduction 6
Preparation Strategies 9
Practice Question 1 11
Practice Question 2 14
Practice Question 3 17
Practice Question 4 20
Practice Question 5 23
Practice Question 6 26
Practice Question 7 28
Practice Question 8 30
Practice Question 9 32
Practice Question 10 34
Practice Question 11 36
Practice Question 12 38
Practice Question 13 40
Practice Question 14 42
Practice Question 15 44
Practice Question 16 47
Practice Question 17 50
Practice Question 18 52
Practice Question 19 55

Practice Question 20 58
Practice Question 21 61
Practice Question 22 64
Practice Question 23 67
Practice Question 24 70
Practice Question 25 73
Practice Question 26 76
Practice Question 27 79
Practice Question 28 82
Practice Question 29 85
Practice Question 30 87
Practice Question 31 90
Practice Question 32 93
Practice Question 33 95
Practice Question 34 98
Practice Question 35 101
Practice Question 36 104
Practice Question 37 107
Practice Question 38 110
Practice Question 39 113
Practice Question 40 116
Practice Question 41 119
Practice Question 42 121
Practice Question 43 123

Practice Question 44 126
Practice Question 45 129
Practice Question 46 132
Practice Question 47 135
Practice Question 48 138
Practice Question 49 141
Practice Question 50 144
Practice Question 51 147
Practice Question 52 149
Practice Question 53 152
Practice Question 54 155
Practice Question 55 158
Practice Question 56 161
Practice Question 57 164
Practice Question 58 167
Practice Question 59 170
Practice Question 60 173

Introduction

When aspiring to the medical profession, preparation is crucial. The recent emergence of the AAMC PREview exam in the medical school application process means future doctors must understand its significance and strategies to tackle it.

In this book we will introduce the AAMC PREview exam, provide some tips, and then jump right in to 60 practice scenarios with model answers so that you understand how to ace the AAMC PREview exam!

Before we begin, it is important to note that this publication and its content are not affiliated with, endorsed by, or sponsored by the Association of American Medical Colleges (AAMC) or any official AAMC exam. The practice scenarios and model answers provided in this book are created by the authors and are intended for preparatory purposes only. All trademarks, brand names, and logos mentioned within this book are the property of their respective owners and are used here for identification purposes only. Readers should consult the official AAMC resources and website for definitive guidance and information related to the actual exams.

Why the PREview Exam Matters

The AAMC PREview professional readiness exam, previously the AAMC Situational Judgment Test (SJT), was introduced in the 2020-2021 application cycle. Designed to assess a candidate's professional competence and personal qualities, this test provides a more holistic view of an applicant beyond academic achievements. With the growing emphasis on this exam in the admissions process, it's imperative to be well-prepared.

Not all schools require you to have this as part of your application, so make sure to review your school's requirements carefully. You can view a list of participating schools on the AAMC website.

A Closer Look at AAMC PREview Exam

Structure: The exam presents scenario sets reflecting real-life situations that you may encounter as a future medical student. After each scenario, you will be asked to rate possible actions on a 4 point scale based on their effectiveness:

1 = Very ineffective. "The response will cause additional problems or make the situation worse."

2 = Ineffective. "The response will not improve the situation or may cause a problem."

3 = Effective. "The response could help but will not significantly improve the situation."

4 = Very effective. "The response will significantly help the situation."

It is important to note that you can **use an option more than once for the same scenario**. So, for example, if you are presented with 5 possible actions after a scenario, you could rate them all as Effective (3). This will become clearer as you go through our sample scenarios and model answers.

Scoring: Your answers will be compared to "model answers" which are determined by a panel of medical educators. The closer your answers are to the model answer, the higher your score. There are 30 scenarios on the exam and at end your score is tallied up on a 9 point scale (9 being the highest) relative to other test-takers.

What is measured on the AAMC PREview exam?

The exam assesses for eight core pre-professional competencies for entering medical students:

- Service Orientation.
- Social Skills.
- Cultural Competence.
- Teamwork.
- Ethical Responsibility to Self and Others.
- Resilience and Adaptability.
- Reliability and Dependability.
- Capacity for Improvement.

Preparation Strategies

Review Official AAMC Materials: Start with the AAMC PREview Essentials Guide, providing in-depth details about the exam. The Examinee Preparation Guide is another great resource with sample scenarios and responses. All of these resources can be found on the AAMC website.

Understand the Core Competencies: Dive deep into the eight competencies assessed. Reflect on their importance in the medical field.

Practice: Regularly engage with sample scenarios. Analyze each situation carefully, and always be open-minded. We have you covered on this one! Discussing scenarios with peers can also offer fresh perspectives.

Tips for Exam Day

Technical Setup: Ensure your tech (webcam, microphone, browser) meets the requirements.

Environment: Choose a quiet, well-lit room. Clear your desk, and make sure no distractions are around.

Stay Informed: Understand all exam rules to prevent unexpected interruptions. Your proctor will be monitoring, so stay compliant!

Now it's time to practice!

Practice Question 1

During a clinical rotation, you witness a fellow medical student, Jamie, struggling to draw blood from a patient. The patient is becoming increasingly anxious. The supervising physician is not present in the room.

Please rate the effectiveness of each response to this situation.

1. Stand by quietly, waiting to see if Jamie eventually succeeds, to avoid adding more pressure.
2. Offer gentle suggestions or guidance to Jamie, based on your previous successful experiences.
3. Interrupt and take over from Jamie, assuring the patient you're more skilled.
4. After the session, ask Jamie if they would like to practice together or share some resources that helped you.
5. Tell the patient that Jamie is still learning and they should be patient.

Answer Key & Explanations for Practice Question 1

Stand by quietly, waiting to see if Jamie eventually succeeds, to avoid adding more pressure.
Ineffective (2): While it might seem considerate not to put Jamie on the spot, the patient's well-being and comfort should be the priority. The passive approach might prolong the patient's discomfort.

Offer gentle suggestions or guidance to Jamie, based on your previous successful experiences.
Very Effective (4): Offering assistance in a non-confrontational manner can both support Jamie and reassure the patient.

Interrupt and take over from Jamie, assuring the patient you're more skilled.
Very Ineffective (1): Interrupting Jamie can undermine their confidence and can also be perceived as arrogant, potentially affecting team dynamics.

After the session, ask Jamie if they would like to practice together or share some resources that helped you.
Very Effective (4): Offering help in private, away from the patient, is supportive and fosters a collaborative learning environment.

Tell the patient that Jamie is still learning and they should be patient.

Ineffective (2): While transparency is important, this might increase the patient's anxiety and make Jamie feel more self-conscious.

Practice Question 2

You're in a study group with four other medical students preparing for an important exam. One member, Alex, consistently dominates the discussion and often dismisses others' contributions. The group's productivity is suffering, and members are expressing their frustrations privately.

Please rate the effectiveness of each response to this situation.

1. Publicly confront Alex during the next study session about their behavior.
2. Privately speak to Alex, expressing your concerns and suggesting ways to ensure everyone gets a chance to contribute.
3. Send an anonymous note to Alex addressing their behavior.
4. Propose a study group "round-robin" structure where each member gets dedicated time to speak and share their insights.
5. Avoid future study sessions and study alone to avoid the conflict.

Answer Key & Explanations for Practice Question 2

Publicly confront Alex during the next study session about their behavior.
Ineffective (2): While addressing the issue is important, doing so publicly can embarrass Alex and might create further tension in the group.

Privately speak to Alex, expressing your concerns and suggesting ways to ensure everyone gets a chance to contribute.
Very Effective (4): Addressing the issue privately and in a constructive manner respects Alex's feelings while aiming for a positive resolution.

Send an anonymous note to Alex addressing their behavior.
Very Ineffective (1): An anonymous note can come across as passive-aggressive, and Alex might feel attacked or isolated without knowing how to address or rectify the situation.

Propose a study group "round-robin" structure where each member gets dedicated time to speak and share their insights.
Effective (3): Implementing a structure can ensure everyone gets a chance to speak, but it may not address the root cause of Alex's behavior.

Avoid future study sessions and study alone to avoid the conflict.
Ineffective (2): Avoiding the issue doesn't resolve it and you lose out on the potential benefits of group study.

Practice Question 3

You're in a clinical rotation and are shadowing Dr. Smith, a seasoned physician. During a consultation with a patient, you notice Dr. Smith overlooks a significant detail from the patient's medical history, potentially impacting the diagnosis. The patient seems unaware, and Dr. Smith is moving forward with the treatment recommendation.

Please rate the effectiveness of each response to this situation.

1. Interrupt the consultation immediately to point out the oversight to Dr. Smith.
2. After the consultation, discreetly share your observation with Dr. Smith and ask for clarity.
3. Discuss your observation with fellow medical students to get their opinion on the situation.
4. Make a personal note of the oversight and ensure not to make such mistakes in your future practice, but don't address it with Dr. Smith.
5. Approach the patient privately and inform them of the oversight.

Answer Key & Explanations for Practice Question 3

Interrupt the consultation immediately to point out the oversight to Dr. Smith.
Ineffective (2): Interrupting can disrupt the flow of the consultation and potentially undermine Dr. Smith's authority in front of the patient.

After the consultation, discreetly share your observation with Dr. Smith and ask for clarity.
Very Effective (4): Addressing the issue privately and constructively allows for potential rectification without undermining Dr. Smith in front of the patient.

Discuss your observation with fellow medical students to get their opinion on the situation.
Ineffective (2): While it's helpful to seek peers' opinions, it doesn't directly address the potential risk to the patient's health from the oversight.

Make a personal note of the oversight and ensure not to make such mistakes in your future practice, but don't address it with Dr. Smith.
Ineffective (2): While it's important for personal learning, not addressing the oversight can lead to potential harm for the patient.

Approach the patient privately and inform them of the oversight.

Very Ineffective (1): This action can undermine the trust between the patient and Dr. Smith, potentially leading to legal and ethical complications.

Practice Question 4

During a study session, a fellow medical student, Alex, shares that they have access to exam questions for the upcoming test. Alex offers to show them to you, believing it could help both of you secure better grades.

Please rate the effectiveness of each response to this situation.

1. Agree to see the questions, rationalizing that it's just for preparation and you won't use them during the actual exam.
2. Politely decline Alex's offer and express your discomfort with the situation.
3. Report Alex's behavior to a faculty member or the appropriate authority.
4. Suggest to Alex that studying together without the questions would be more beneficial and ethical.
5. Tell other classmates about the offer to gauge their opinions on the matter.

Answer Key & Explanations for Practice Question 4

Agree to see the questions, rationalizing that it's just for preparation and you won't use them during the actual exam.
Very Ineffective (1): Viewing the exam questions beforehand is unethical and compromises the integrity of the assessment process.

Politely decline Alex's offer and express your discomfort with the situation.
Very Effective (4): This action maintains your personal integrity and conveys the importance of ethics in academic settings.

Report Alex's behavior to a faculty member or the appropriate authority.
Effective (3): Reporting unethical behavior can help maintain the academic integrity of the institution. However, it may also strain your relationship with Alex, which is why it's rated as effective but not very effective.

Suggest to Alex that studying together without the questions would be more beneficial and ethical.
Very Effective (4): Redirecting to a positive and ethical study method benefits both students without compromising integrity.

Tell other classmates about the offer to gauge their opinions on the matter.
Ineffective (2): Sharing the information further can spread the unethical behavior, and gauging opinions doesn't directly address the core issue.

Practice Question 5

You're working on a group project in your medical school program. One of your group members, Jordan, has consistently missed meetings and hasn't contributed much to the project. The project's deadline is approaching, and you're concerned about the potential impact on your grade.

Please rate the effectiveness of each response to this situation.

1. Confront Jordan aggressively about their lack of contribution in front of the entire group.
2. Send Jordan a private message expressing your concerns and asking if everything is okay.
3. Complete Jordan's portion of the project yourself without discussing it with them.
4. Discuss the issue with the whole team to figure out a way to evenly distribute the workload.
5. Request a meeting with the course instructor to discuss Jordan's contribution.

Answer Key & Explanations for Practice Question 5

Confront Jordan aggressively about their lack of contribution in front of the entire group.
Very Ineffective (1): Aggressively confronting a team member in front of others can lead to unnecessary tension and conflicts within the group.

Send Jordan a private message expressing your concerns and asking if everything is okay.
Very Effective (4): Approaching Jordan in a non-confrontational manner gives them an opportunity to explain their situation and possibly find a solution.

Complete Jordan's portion of the project yourself without discussing it with them.
Ineffective (2): While it may ensure the project gets done, it doesn't address the root issue and might lead to resentment or misunderstanding.

Discuss the issue with the whole team to figure out a way to evenly distribute the workload.
Effective (3): Collaboration can lead to solutions, but it's essential to approach the situation in a constructive way without singling out or blaming Jordan.

Request a meeting with the course instructor to discuss Jordan's contribution.
Effective (3): It's a proactive approach, but it's essential to ensure you've tried other avenues first. Going directly to the

instructor might be seen as escalating the situation prematurely.

Practice Question 6

While studying for an important upcoming exam, you discover a group of students sharing answers to a practice test that they obtained from a previous year, which is against the school's academic integrity policies. You know a couple of these students personally.

Please rate the effectiveness of each response to this situation.

1. Ignore the situation and focus on your own studies without getting involved.
2. Confront the group of students and ask them to stop sharing the answers.
3. Report the incident to the course instructor or the appropriate academic authority.
4. Discuss your concerns with a trusted peer or mentor before deciding on any action.
5. Offer to organize a legitimate study group to help everyone prepare better for the exam.

Answer Key & Explanations for Practice Question 6

Ignore the situation and focus on your own studies without getting involved.
Ineffective (2): While it avoids conflict, it doesn't address the breach of academic integrity.

Confront the group of students and ask them to stop sharing the answers.
Effective (3): Directly addressing the issue can be a good approach, but it may lead to confrontations. It's essential to approach with care.

Report the incident to the course instructor or the appropriate academic authority.
Very Effective (4): Upholding the school's academic integrity policies is crucial. Reporting ensures that the issue is handled appropriately.

Discuss your concerns with a trusted peer or mentor before deciding on any action.
Effective (3): Seeking advice can offer a balanced perspective and might help you decide the best course of action.

Offer to organize a legitimate study group to help everyone prepare better for the exam.
Effective (3): Promoting honest academic practices and helping peers is a positive step, though it doesn't directly address the cheating issue.

Practice Question 7

You are assigned to a group project with four other students. As the deadline approaches, you notice one member, Alex, hasn't contributed as much as the others. During a meeting, another group member confronts Alex about their lack of contribution in a rather aggressive manner.

Please rate the effectiveness of each response to this situation.

1. Allow the confrontation to continue, hoping it will motivate Alex to contribute more.
2. Suggest a short break, then privately ask Alex if there's a reason for their reduced contribution.
3. Immediately defend Alex, pointing out the times they did contribute.
4. Calmly intervene, suggesting the group discusses workload distribution and how to support each other better.
5. Propose that the group divides Alex's unfinished tasks among the other members without further discussion.

Answer Key & Explanations for Practice Question 7

Allow the confrontation to continue, hoping it will motivate Alex to contribute more.
Ineffective (2): Letting conflicts escalate can harm group dynamics and may not result in the desired outcome.

Suggest a short break, then privately ask Alex if there's a reason for their reduced contribution.
Very Effective (4): By addressing the issue privately, you can understand any underlying reasons and potentially find a solution without causing further embarrassment or tension.

Immediately defend Alex, pointing out the times they did contribute.
Effective (3): While defending a team member can be positive, it might not address the core issue or solve the problem.

Calmly intervene, suggesting the group discusses workload distribution and how to support each other better.
Very Effective (4): Promoting open dialogue can help understand everyone's concerns and work towards a collective solution.

Propose that the group divides Alex's unfinished tasks among the other members without further discussion.
Effective (3): While this may help in the short term to get the project done, it doesn't address the underlying issues or ensure equal contribution from all members.

Practice Question 8

You are in your second year of medical school and have been consistently performing well. A first-year student, Jordan, approaches you for advice on managing stress and time, as they're struggling with their workload.

Please rate the effectiveness of each response to this situation.

1. Tell Jordan that medical school is meant to be challenging and they should just push through.
2. Share with Jordan some of the study techniques and relaxation methods that have worked for you.
3. Recommend to Jordan to consider if medical school is the right path for them.
4. Organize a study group where Jordan can join and learn from peers.
5. Suggest Jordan meet with an academic counselor to discuss their challenges and seek guidance.

Answer Key & Explanations for Practice Question 8

Tell Jordan that medical school is meant to be challenging and they should just push through.
Ineffective (2): While medical school is challenging, this response may come off as dismissive and may not be helpful to Jordan.

Share with Jordan some of the study techniques and relaxation methods that have worked for you.
Very Effective (4): Providing practical advice based on personal experience can be beneficial and supportive.

Recommend to Jordan to consider if medical school is the right path for them.
Ineffective (2): Although well-intended, this could demotivate Jordan and make them feel more isolated.

Organize a study group where Jordan can join and learn from peers.
Very Effective (4): Peer learning can be beneficial, and it can also foster a sense of community and belonging.

Suggest Jordan meet with an academic counselor to discuss their challenges and seek guidance.
Very Effective (4): Seeking professional guidance can offer tailored strategies and resources that can assist Jordan in their academic journey.

Practice Question 9

During a clinical rotation, you overhear a colleague making an inappropriate comment about a patient's background. The patient seems unaware, but you're uncomfortable with what was said.

Please rate the effectiveness of each response to this situation.

1. Ignore the comment and focus on your tasks to avoid any confrontation.
2. Report the incident to a supervisor or someone in a position of authority without confronting the colleague.
3. Approach the colleague privately and express your concerns about their comment.
4. Discuss the situation with other peers to get their opinion on what to do.
5. Address the comment immediately in front of the patient and colleague, expressing your discomfort.

Answer Key & Explanations for Practice Question 9

Ignore the comment and focus on your tasks to avoid any confrontation.
Ineffective (2): Ignoring such situations can perpetuate a culture of insensitivity and could compromise patient care and trust.

Report the incident to a supervisor or someone in a position of authority without confronting the colleague.
Effective (3): Reporting ensures that the situation is handled properly, but discussing it with the colleague might also be beneficial to prevent such incidents in the future.

Approach the colleague privately and express your concerns about their comment.
Very Effective (4): Addressing the issue directly can lead to understanding and change without escalating the situation.

Discuss the situation with other peers to get their opinion on what to do.
Effective (3): Seeking advice can provide perspective, but it's important to ensure that the situation is handled appropriately and not just become a topic of gossip.

Address the comment immediately in front of the patient and colleague, expressing your discomfort.
Ineffective (2): This could escalate the situation and make the patient feel even more uncomfortable or singled out.

Practice Question 10

You are on a group project with three other medical students. Two of the members, including you, have been contributing regularly to the project. However, one member hasn't shown up to any meetings or contributed to the work. The deadline is approaching.

Please rate the effectiveness of each response to this situation.

1. Complete the project with the contributing members and mark the non-contributing member's name off the final submission.
2. Email the non-contributing member, expressing your concerns about their lack of participation and asking if there's any reason for it.
3. Submit a complaint to the course coordinator about the non-contributing member without talking to them.
4. Approach the non-contributing member in person and discuss ways they can contribute before the deadline.
5. Discuss the situation with the other contributing member and decide on a collective course of action.

Answer Key & Explanations for Practice Question 10

Complete the project with the contributing members and mark the non-contributing member's name off the final submission.
Ineffective (2): Without communication, this can lead to misunderstandings and potential conflicts.

Email the non-contributing member, expressing your concerns about their lack of participation and asking if there's any reason for it.
Effective (3): Addressing the issue and offering a chance for the member to explain their situation is a balanced approach.

Submit a complaint to the course coordinator about the non-contributing member without talking to them.
Ineffective (2): It's better to address concerns directly before involving higher authorities.

Approach the non-contributing member in person and discuss ways they can contribute before the deadline.
Very Effective (4): This direct and constructive approach promotes teamwork and gives the non-contributing member a chance to rectify their behavior.

Discuss the situation with the other contributing member and decide on a collective course of action.
Effective (3): Collective decision-making ensures all stakeholders are on the same page and can lead to a more unified solution.

Practice Question 11

While on rounds in the hospital, you overhear a fellow medical student discussing a patient's private health information loudly in the elevator, where others not involved in the patient's care can hear.

Please rate the effectiveness of each response to this situation.

1. Address the medical student privately, reminding them of the importance of patient confidentiality.
2. Immediately interrupt the student in the elevator, pointing out their mistake.
3. Report the student to the supervising physician without speaking to the student first.
4. Discuss the incident in a group setting with other medical students to see if they've noticed similar behavior.
5. Ignore the incident, assuming the student will eventually learn the importance of privacy.

Answer Key & Explanations for Practice Question 11

Address the medical student privately, reminding them of the importance of patient confidentiality.
Very Effective (4): Addressing the issue privately respects the student's dignity while emphasizing the importance of confidentiality.

Immediately interrupt the student in the elevator, pointing out their mistake.
Effective (3): Although it stops the breach in confidentiality, it may embarrass the student in front of others.

Report the student to the supervising physician without speaking to the student first.
Ineffective (2): Direct communication with the student should be attempted before escalating to superiors.

Discuss the incident in a group setting with other medical students to see if they've noticed similar behavior.
Ineffective (2): This may lead to gossip or unwanted negative attention towards the student without addressing the root of the issue.

Ignore the incident, assuming the student will eventually learn the importance of privacy.
Very Ineffective (1): Patient confidentiality is paramount, and ignoring breaches can lead to further incidents and potential harm.

Practice Question 12

You are part of a study group, and one of the members consistently arrives late, disrupting the flow of the study session. Other members have expressed their frustration to you privately.

Please rate the effectiveness of each response to this situation.

1. Decide to change the group's meeting time without informing the latecomer.
2. Confront the late member publicly during the next session about their tardiness.
3. Have a private conversation with the late member to understand their reasons and discuss potential solutions.
4. Disband the study group without explaining why.
5. Start the session on time regardless and catch the late member up during breaks.

Answer Key & Explanations for Practice Question 12

Decide to change the group's meeting time without informing the latecomer.
Ineffective (2): This approach is passive-aggressive and doesn't directly address the issue or give the late member an opportunity to rectify the situation.

Confront the late member publicly during the next session about their tardiness.
Ineffective (2): Public confrontation can lead to embarrassment and defensiveness, hindering a constructive resolution.

Have a private conversation with the late member to understand their reasons and discuss potential solutions.
Very Effective (4): Direct and respectful communication provides an opportunity for understanding and collaboration, leading to potential solutions.

Disband the study group without explaining why.
Very Ineffective (1): This drastic action punishes all members and avoids addressing the specific issue, denying the group the potential benefits of studying together.

Start the session on time regardless and catch the late member up during breaks.
Effective (3): This maintains the group's productivity, though it may not directly address the root cause of the tardiness.

Practice Question 13

During a clinical rotation, you notice that one of your peers is not following the correct handwashing protocols before interacting with patients, potentially putting patients at risk.

Please rate the effectiveness of each response to this situation.

1. Ignore the situation since it's not your responsibility.
2. Inform the supervising physician immediately without speaking to your peer.
3. Pull your peer aside and discuss the importance of following the handwashing protocols, providing them with resources if necessary.
4. Talk about your peer's negligence during lunch breaks with other students without addressing it directly with them.
5. Offer to practice the correct handwashing technique together after the rotation.

Answer Key & Explanations for Practice Question 13

Ignore the situation since it's not your responsibility.
Ineffective (2): Patient safety should be everyone's priority, and ignoring it could lead to potential harm.

Inform the supervising physician immediately without speaking to your peer.
Effective (3): While it is essential to ensure patient safety, direct communication with the peer might have resolved the issue without escalating it.

Pull your peer aside and discuss the importance of following the handwashing protocols, providing them with resources if necessary.
Very Effective (4): Addressing the issue directly with your peer in a constructive manner allows for understanding and rectification of behavior.

Talk about your peer's negligence during lunch breaks with other students without addressing it directly with them.
Very Ineffective (1): This approach is unprofessional, doesn't address the issue, and might lead to creating an unwarranted negative reputation for your peer.

Offer to practice the correct handwashing technique together after the rotation.
Effective (3): This friendly approach could make your peer more receptive and aware, though it's more passive and might delay addressing the immediate concern.

Practice Question 14

You're in a study group, and one of the members consistently comes late, distracting others and causing delays in starting the study sessions. This has led to frustration among the group members.

Please rate the effectiveness of each response to this situation.

1. Address the issue in the group chat without mentioning the late member's name, hoping they get the hint.
2. Speak directly to the member, expressing your concerns and understanding if there are reasons for their tardiness.
3. Complain about the member to others outside of the study group.
4. Start the study session on time, irrespective of whether this member has arrived.
5. Consider changing the study group's timings, discussing it with everyone, including the consistently late member.

Answer Key & Explanations for Practice Question 14

Address the issue in the group chat without mentioning the late member's name, hoping they get the hint.
Ineffective (2): Indirect communication might not be understood or may come across as passive-aggressive, creating a negative atmosphere.

Speak directly to the member, expressing your concerns and understanding if there are reasons for their tardiness.
Very Effective (4): Direct communication is often the best approach to resolve issues, as it allows for understanding and finding solutions.

Complain about the member to others outside of the study group.
Very Ineffective (1): Complaining doesn't address the issue and can strain relationships within and outside of the group.

Start the study session on time, irrespective of whether this member has arrived.
Effective (3): It ensures the group's study time isn't compromised, but it may not address the root issue of tardiness.

Consider changing the study group's timings, discussing it with everyone, including the consistently late member.
Effective (3): While this is a considerate approach, it might not be feasible for everyone and could be seen as accommodating one person's needs over the group's.

Practice Question 15

You have been paired with a classmate for a joint project. As the deadline approaches, you realize that your partner has not contributed equally, leaving most of the work to you.

Please rate the effectiveness of each response to this situation.

1. Complete the project on your own without communicating your concerns to your partner.
2. Address the issue with your partner, discussing a plan for equal contribution moving forward.
3. Report the issue to your professor without discussing it with your partner first.
4. Propose a clear division of the remaining tasks and set deadlines for each.
5. Avoid future group projects with this classmate without addressing the current situation.

Answer Key & Explanations for Practice Question 15

Complete the project on your own without communicating your concerns to your partner.
Ineffective (2): While it ensures the project's completion, it doesn't address the unequal contribution or give your partner a chance to rectify the situation.

Address the issue with your partner, discussing a plan for equal contribution moving forward.
Very Effective (4): This approach fosters communication, allows for understanding, and provides a path forward for both parties.

Report the issue to your professor without discussing it with your partner first.
Ineffective (2): It's generally better to try and resolve the issue between yourselves first, as escalation might strain the relationship without giving a chance for resolution.

Propose a clear division of the remaining tasks and set deadlines for each.
Effective (3): It offers a structured way to handle the remainder of the project, though it might still be seen as reactive rather than addressing the root issue.

Avoid future group projects with this classmate without addressing the current situation.
Ineffective (2): While this avoids future complications, it doesn't address the immediate issue or give room for growth in the relationship.

Practice Question 16

During a patient round, you observe a senior resident making a potential mistake in a patient's medication dose. The resident has not noticed their error, and the attending physician is not present.

Please rate the effectiveness of each response to this situation.

1. Quietly correct the error without informing the senior resident.
2. Immediately bring it to the senior resident's attention in a respectful manner.
3. Discuss your observation with your peers to get their opinion before taking action.
4. Wait for the attending physician to return and inform them of the mistake.
5. Document the error without confronting the senior resident or informing any supervising authority.

Answer Key & Explanations for Practice Question 16

Quietly correct the error without informing the senior resident.
Ineffective (2): While it addresses the immediate issue, it does not provide the senior resident with the opportunity to learn and could lead to further errors in the future.

Immediately bring it to the senior resident's attention in a respectful manner.
Very Effective (4): This approach is proactive, promotes learning, and ensures patient safety without causing unnecessary conflict.

Discuss your observation with your peers to get their opinion before taking action.
Ineffective (2): While seeking peer input can be valuable, time-sensitive matters like potential medication errors should be addressed immediately to ensure patient safety.

Wait for the attending physician to return and inform them of the mistake.
Effective (3): While it's good to involve a higher authority, waiting could put the patient at risk if the medication is administered before the attending physician is informed.

Document the error without confronting the senior resident or informing any supervising authority.

Very Ineffective (1): Merely documenting without acting could lead to serious harm to the patient, and it misses an opportunity for corrective feedback.

Practice Question 17

You're in a study group preparing for an upcoming exam. One of the group members consistently dominates the discussion and rarely gives others a chance to speak. This is making it difficult for everyone to participate and benefit from the group.

Please rate the effectiveness of each response to this situation.

1. Stay silent and hope the group member realizes their behavior on their own.
2. Discuss the issue privately with the group member after the session.
3. Publicly confront the group member during the session about their behavior.
4. Suggest a round-robin approach where each member gets a turn to speak.
5. Disband the study group without addressing the issue.

Answer Key & Explanations for Practice Question 17

Stay silent and hope the group member realizes their behavior on their own.
Ineffective (2): Passive approaches rarely solve issues, and there's no guarantee the group member will recognize their behavior without feedback.

Discuss the issue privately with the group member after the session.
Effective (3): Addressing the issue privately avoids public confrontation, but it's possible that the group member might become defensive.

Publicly confront the group member during the session about their behavior.
Ineffective (2): While direct, this approach might lead to defensiveness or conflict, further disrupting the group dynamic.

Suggest a round-robin approach where each member gets a turn to speak.
Very Effective (4): This is a proactive, structured solution that ensures everyone gets a chance to participate without directly confronting the dominating group member.

Disband the study group without addressing the issue.
Very Ineffective (1): Avoiding the problem entirely deprives everyone of the potential benefits of the study group.

Practice Question 18

You are shadowing a doctor in the emergency department when you witness a nurse being rude to a patient. The patient is visibly upset by the interaction. You're unsure of the hospital's protocols in such situations.

Please rate the effectiveness of each response to this situation.

1. Immediately confront the nurse about their behavior in front of the patient.
2. Discuss the situation privately with the doctor you are shadowing for guidance.
3. Apologize to the patient on behalf of the nurse without discussing it with the nurse.
4. Document the incident and report it to the hospital's ethics committee.
5. Talk to the nurse privately and express your concerns about the interaction.

Answer Key & Explanations for Practice Question 18

Immediately confront the nurse about their behavior in front of the patient.
Ineffective (2): While it's important to address issues, confronting a colleague in front of a patient might escalate the situation and isn't professional.

Discuss the situation privately with the doctor you are shadowing for guidance.
Very Effective (4): As a student, seeking guidance from someone more experienced is a wise step, especially when unsure of protocols.

Apologize to the patient on behalf of the nurse without discussing it with the nurse.
Effective (3): Empathizing with the patient is important, but it's also essential to address the root cause with the nurse or through proper channels.

Document the incident and report it to the hospital's ethics committee.
Effective (3): Reporting inappropriate behavior is essential, but as a shadow, understanding the hospital's protocol first is crucial.

Talk to the nurse privately and express your concerns about the interaction.

Effective (3): Addressing concerns directly can lead to understanding and resolution, but as a student, it's essential to approach with humility and a desire to learn.

Practice Question 19

During a study group session, one of your peers, who usually excels academically, confesses to feeling overwhelmed and considers dropping out of medical school. They mention not being able to handle the stress and pressure anymore.

Please rate the effectiveness of each response to this situation.

1. Tell your peer that everyone feels stressed, and they just need to push through it.
2. Offer to help them with their studies and suggest relaxation techniques.
3. Encourage your peer to speak with a school counselor or professional about their feelings.
4. Share your own experiences of feeling overwhelmed, empathizing with their situation.
5. Advise them to take a break from medical school if they feel it's too much.

Answer Key & Explanations for Practice Question 19

Tell your peer that everyone feels stressed, and they just need to push through it.
Ineffective (2): While many students feel stress, dismissing or minimizing their feelings isn't constructive or supportive.

Offer to help them with their studies and suggest relaxation techniques.
Effective (3): Lending a hand academically and suggesting coping mechanisms can be helpful, but it might not address the root cause of their distress.

Encourage your peer to speak with a school counselor or professional about their feelings.
Very Effective (4): Recommending professional help ensures that they receive guidance tailored to their unique struggles, addressing both emotional and academic concerns.

Share your own experiences of feeling overwhelmed, empathizing with their situation.
Effective (3): Sharing personal experiences can create a bond and offer comfort in knowing they aren't alone, but it's also vital to ensure they get the proper help they need.

Advise them to take a break from medical school if they feel it's too much.
Ineffective (2): While a break might help, it's essential to consider the long-term implications and other options first.

It's best for them to make such a decision with the guidance of professionals.

Practice Question 20

You are participating in a group project, and one of the group members consistently misses deadlines, causing delays for everyone else. The final presentation is due in a week, and the group's grade heavily depends on this project.

Please rate the effectiveness of each response to this situation.

1. Decide to take over the absent group member's tasks without discussing it with the group.
2. Arrange a group meeting to discuss the issue and come up with a plan to manage the workload.
3. Email the professor explaining the situation and asking for an extension.
4. Confront the group member privately, asking about their absences and if they need assistance.
5. Assign all the remaining tasks to the non-participating member, ensuring they catch up on their part.

Answer Key & Explanations for Practice Question 20

Decide to take over the absent group member's tasks without discussing it with the group.
Ineffective (2): Taking unilateral decisions without discussing with the group can lead to misunderstandings and further group dynamics issues.

Arrange a group meeting to discuss the issue and come up with a plan to manage the workload.
Very Effective (4): Open communication with all group members can help find a solution collectively, ensuring everyone is on the same page.

Email the professor explaining the situation and asking for an extension.
Effective (3): While communicating with the professor is essential, it might be best to try solving the issue within the group first before seeking external solutions.

Confront the group member privately, asking about their absences and if they need assistance.
Effective (3): Addressing the issue directly can help in understanding the reasons behind the consistent absence and offer a way to provide support if needed.

Assign all the remaining tasks to the non-participating member, ensuring they catch up on their part.
Ineffective (2): Overloading the non-participating member without understanding their situation can lead to more delays and possible resentment.

Practice Question 21

During your clinical rotations, you notice a fellow medical student consistently being disrespectful towards nurses. This has started to affect the team dynamics, with nurses being hesitant to interact with students.

Please rate the effectiveness of each response to this situation.

1. Ignore the behavior, assuming that someone else will address it.
2. Approach the fellow student privately, expressing your observations and concerns.
3. Talk negatively about the fellow student's behavior with other medical students.
4. Report the behavior to a senior doctor or supervisor without discussing it with the student.
5. Encourage a meeting between the student, nurses, and a mediator to address and resolve the issue.

Answer Key & Explanations for Practice Question 21

Ignore the behavior, assuming that someone else will address it.
Ineffective (2): Ignoring problematic behavior can perpetuate it and might damage team dynamics even more over time.

Approach the fellow student privately, expressing your observations and concerns.
Very Effective (4): Addressing the issue directly with the individual can lead to a better understanding, and they might not be aware of the impact of their behavior.

Talk negatively about the fellow student's behavior with other medical students.
Very Ineffective (1): This can lead to further damage to the reputation of the student, exacerbate team issues, and does not provide a solution to the problem.

Report the behavior to a senior doctor or supervisor without discussing it with the student.
Effective (3): Reporting to a higher authority might be necessary in certain situations, but discussing the matter with the individual first can sometimes lead to a resolution without escalation.

Encourage a meeting between the student, nurses, and a mediator to address and resolve the issue.
Very Effective (4): Encouraging open communication and resolving misunderstandings with a neutral party can restore team dynamics and ensure a healthy working environment.

Practice Question 22

You're working on a group project with three other medical students. Two of the students have taken on a majority of the work, leaving you and the fourth student with very little contribution. The fourth student suggests that you both just let the other two handle everything since they seem to have it under control.

Please rate the effectiveness of each response to this situation.

1. Agree with the fourth student and let the other two students do the entire project.
2. Speak with all group members and discuss how tasks can be redistributed for everyone to have an equal share.
3. Complete another portion of the project without discussing it with anyone and submit it as your contribution.
4. Confront the two students who took over, accusing them of trying to dominate the group.
5. Ask the two active students if they need any assistance or if there's any part of the project you can help with.

Answer Key & Explanations for Practice Question 22

Agree with the fourth student and let the other two students do the entire project.
Ineffective (2): Not contributing to a group project is unfair to those who are putting in the effort and doesn't showcase your commitment to the task.

Speak with all group members and discuss how tasks can be redistributed for everyone to have an equal share.
Very Effective (4): Open communication can help in ensuring everyone has an opportunity to contribute equally. It addresses the issue constructively.

Complete another portion of the project without discussing it with anyone and submit it as your contribution.
Ineffective (2): Working without coordination can lead to redundancy and might not be in line with what the group needs.

Confront the two students who took over, accusing them of trying to dominate the group.
Very Ineffective (1): Confrontation without understanding their perspective can lead to further conflicts and is not a productive approach.

Ask the two active students if they need any assistance or if there's any part of the project you can help with.

Very Effective (4): Offering help showcases your commitment and ensures that you're actively participating while also understanding their perspective.

Practice Question 23

You're in a clinical rotation and one of your patients, an elderly gentleman, consistently refuses to take his medications. He claims they make him feel "foggy" and insists he's better off without them. Your attending physician is becoming frustrated with the patient's non-compliance.

Please rate the effectiveness of each response to this situation.

1. Tell the patient that if he doesn't take his medications, there's nothing more the medical team can do for him.
2. Patiently ask the patient to explain his concerns in detail, ensuring he feels heard and understood.
3. Discuss the patient's concerns with the attending physician and ask if there are alternative treatments or approaches that could be considered.
4. Inform the patient that refusing medications could have severe consequences and he should follow medical advice.
5. Share with the patient stories of other patients who suffered due to not taking their medications to scare him into compliance.

Answer Key & Explanations for Practice Question 23

Tell the patient that if he doesn't take his medications, there's nothing more the medical team can do for him.
Ineffective (2): This approach might make the patient feel cornered and not supported. It lacks empathy and understanding.

Patiently ask the patient to explain his concerns in detail, ensuring he feels heard and understood.
Very Effective (4): Actively listening to the patient's concerns can lead to better understanding and can help in tailoring the treatment approach that addresses his fears.

Discuss the patient's concerns with the attending physician and ask if there are alternative treatments or approaches that could be considered.
Very Effective (4): Collaborating with the attending physician to find a solution that works best for the patient showcases initiative and concern for the patient's well-being.

Inform the patient that refusing medications could have severe consequences and he should follow medical advice.
Effective (3): While it's important for the patient to understand the implications of not taking his medications, this approach should be combined with understanding and empathy.

Share with the patient stories of other patients who suffered due to not taking their medications to scare him into compliance.

Ineffective (2): Using fear as a tactic might not be the best approach, as it may cause further resistance or mistrust in the patient-doctor relationship.

Practice Question 24

You are in a group study session for a challenging medical school exam. One of the members, Alex, consistently dominates the conversation, asserting that his way of understanding the material is the only correct one. Other group members are becoming frustrated because they feel their viewpoints are being overshadowed.

Please rate the effectiveness of each response to this situation.

1. Confront Alex in front of the group and tell him he's being overbearing.
2. Suggest to the group that everyone should have an equal amount of time to share their thoughts.
3. Stay silent and let Alex continue to dominate the study session.
4. After the session, talk to Alex privately and share the group's feelings, asking if he could allow others to share their insights.
5. Begin to challenge Alex's viewpoints during the study session to undermine his confidence.

Answer Key & Explanations for Practice Question 24

Confront Alex in front of the group and tell him he's being overbearing.

Ineffective (2): Direct confrontation in front of others can cause defensiveness and escalate the situation.

Suggest to the group that everyone should have an equal amount of time to share their thoughts.

Very Effective (4): Implementing a fair structure ensures everyone has an opportunity to contribute, which can mitigate dominance by any single individual.

Stay silent and let Alex continue to dominate the study session.

Very Ineffective (1): This approach doesn't address the issue and allows the group's dynamics to remain unbalanced.

After the session, talk to Alex privately and share the group's feelings, asking if he could allow others to share their insights.

Effective (3): A private conversation can be a diplomatic way to address the issue without causing public confrontation. However, timing matters, and addressing it sooner might be more beneficial.

Begin to challenge Alex's viewpoints during the study session to undermine his confidence.

Ineffective (2): This tactic can lead to unnecessary conflict and does not promote a supportive group learning environment.

Practice Question 25

In the midst of your hectic schedule, you have accidentally double-booked yourself for a patient appointment and a mandatory seminar. Both commitments are of equal importance, and you cannot decide which one to prioritize.

Please rate the effectiveness of each response to this situation.

1. Cancel the patient appointment without giving a reason and attend the seminar.
2. Send an email to the seminar organizer explaining your situation and ask if there is any way to catch up on what you will miss.
3. Attend the patient appointment and ask a colleague to take notes for you during the seminar.
4. Try to reschedule the patient for a time immediately after the seminar.
5. Divide your time by briefly attending the patient appointment and then rush to catch the second half of the seminar.

Answer Key & Explanations for Practice Question 25

Cancel the patient appointment without giving a reason and attend the seminar.
Ineffective (2): Abruptly canceling without providing an explanation can negatively impact the patient's experience and trust in healthcare services.

Send an email to the seminar organizer explaining your situation and ask if there is any way to catch up on what you will miss.
Effective (3): Communicating with the seminar organizer shows responsibility and may provide alternative solutions.

Attend the patient appointment and ask a colleague to take notes for you during the seminar.
Very Effective (4): This solution respects the patient's time and commitment while also ensuring you don't miss out completely on the seminar content.

Try to reschedule the patient for a time immediately after the seminar.
Effective (3): This is a balanced approach, but it depends on the patient's availability and flexibility.

Divide your time by briefly attending the patient appointment and then rush to catch the second half of the seminar.

Ineffective (2): Splitting attention can jeopardize the quality of care provided to the patient and may result in missing critical information from both the appointment and the seminar.

Practice Question 26

While studying in a group, one of your peers frequently belittles others' understanding of the material, causing discomfort among the group members. You've noticed that the group's productivity is decreasing due to the negative atmosphere.

Please rate the effectiveness of each response to this situation.

1. Ignore the negative comments and continue studying as if nothing happened.
2. Privately speak with the peer, expressing your concerns about the negative comments and their impact on the group's productivity.
3. Publicly confront the peer during the study session, challenging them on every negative comment they make.
4. Disband the study group without providing a reason.
5. Ask the group for feedback on how everyone feels about the study sessions, fostering open communication.

Answer Key & Explanations for Practice Question 26

Ignore the negative comments and continue studying as if nothing happened.
Ineffective (2): Ignoring the problem may lead to further deterioration of group dynamics and may not address the root cause of the issue.

Privately speak with the peer, expressing your concerns about the negative comments and their impact on the group's productivity.
Very Effective (4): Addressing the issue privately shows respect for the individual while addressing the behavior that is impacting the group. It provides an opportunity for the peer to understand and modify their behavior.

Publicly confront the peer during the study session, challenging them on every negative comment they make.
Ineffective (2): Confronting the peer publicly might escalate the situation and could cause more discomfort among group members.

Disband the study group without providing a reason.
Very Ineffective (1): This does not address the behavior of the individual causing the problem and penalizes everyone in the group.

Ask the group for feedback on how everyone feels about the study sessions, fostering open communication.

Effective (3): Encouraging open communication can help identify problems and potentially lead to solutions. However, it's essential to ensure that this doesn't turn into a situation where one member feels attacked by the group.

Practice Question 27

You are in a biochemistry lecture, and the professor is explaining a complex pathway. A classmate sitting next to you whispers that they don't understand a specific step. You grasp the concept well and believe you can explain it. The professor is known for not appreciating interruptions during lectures.

Please rate the effectiveness of each response to this situation.

1. Immediately explain the step to your classmate during the lecture.
2. Suggest to your classmate to meet after class so you can explain the concept in detail.
3. Raise your hand and ask the professor to explain the step again for clarification.
4. Tell your classmate to review the textbook or online resources later.
5. Write down a brief explanation on a piece of paper and pass it to your classmate.

Answer Key & Explanations for Practice Question 27

Immediately explain the step to your classmate during the lecture.
Ineffective (2): While it's good to help, speaking during the lecture might distract others and might be seen as disrespectful by the professor.

Suggest to your classmate to meet after class so you can explain the concept in detail.
Very Effective (4): This approach helps your classmate without causing disruption during the lecture.

Raise your hand and ask the professor to explain the step again for clarification.
Effective (3): Asking for clarification can benefit others who might also be confused, but considering the professor's dislike for interruptions, it's essential to gauge the right moment.

Tell your classmate to review the textbook or online resources later.
Ineffective (2): While it's a possible solution, it doesn't immediately help your classmate, and the tone might come off as dismissive.

Write down a brief explanation on a piece of paper and pass it to your classmate.

Effective (3): This method provides an immediate answer without vocal disruption, though passing notes can still be distracting.

Practice Question 28

During a clinical rotation, you observe a senior physician making a potential error in prescribing medication to a patient. The physician is known for being strict and doesn't take feedback well, especially from junior members. However, you are concerned about the patient's well-being.

Please rate the effectiveness of each response to this situation.

1. Immediately confront the senior physician in front of the patient about the error.
2. Wait until after the patient leaves, then discuss your concerns privately with the senior physician.
3. Document the error and report it to the hospital administration without discussing it with the physician.
4. Seek guidance from another senior physician or mentor on how best to address the situation.
5. Stay silent about the incident, considering the senior physician's experience and reputation.

Answer Key & Explanations for Practice Question 28

Immediately confront the senior physician in front of the patient about the error.
Ineffective (2): Addressing the issue immediately may protect the patient, but doing so in front of the patient might undermine the physician's credibility and may not be professionally appropriate.

Wait until after the patient leaves, then discuss your concerns privately with the senior physician.
Very Effective (4): Addressing your concerns privately maintains respect and professionalism while still advocating for the patient's well-being.

Document the error and report it to the hospital administration without discussing it with the physician.
Effective (3): While it's crucial to ensure patient safety, bypassing the physician may escalate the situation unnecessarily if it's an easily rectifiable error.

Seek guidance from another senior physician or mentor on how best to address the situation.
Very Effective (4): Seeking advice from someone experienced can provide a balanced perspective and may help in addressing the issue effectively.

Stay silent about the incident, considering the senior physician's experience and reputation.
Very Ineffective (1): Ignoring potential mistakes, especially those that might harm a patient, is never the right approach, regardless of the seniority or reputation of the physician.

Practice Question 29

You are a medical student in the middle of your rotations, and you are assigned to work with a resident who has a reputation for being particularly demanding and not very patient with students. On your first day, the resident gives you a long list of tasks, some of which you have not been trained to perform yet.

Please rate the effectiveness of each response to this situation.

1. Try to perform all the tasks to the best of your ability, even if you're unsure about some of them.
2. Speak to the resident and clarify which tasks you are trained to perform and ask for guidance on the others.
3. Discuss the situation with your supervising attending physician without informing the resident.
4. Avoid the tasks you're unfamiliar with and only focus on those you know.
5. Request a different resident to work with due to the mismatch in expectations.

Answer Key & Explanations for Practice Question 29

Try to perform all the tasks to the best of your ability, even if you're unsure about some of them.
Ineffective (2): While showing initiative is good, performing tasks without proper training can lead to errors and jeopardize patient safety.

Speak to the resident and clarify which tasks you are trained to perform and ask for guidance on the others.
Very Effective (4): Open communication is crucial. Asking for guidance not only ensures that tasks are performed correctly but also shows your commitment to learning.

Discuss the situation with your supervising attending physician without informing the resident.
Effective (3): While it's essential to seek guidance when feeling overwhelmed, it might be more productive to first communicate directly with the resident about your concerns.

Avoid the tasks you're unfamiliar with and only focus on those you know.
Ineffective (2): Ignoring tasks without communicating why might give the impression of neglecting responsibilities.

Request a different resident to work with due to the mismatch in expectations.
Ineffective (2): Switching residents without attempting communication may not address the underlying issues, and it might not be feasible in all situations.

Practice Question 30

During your medical school rotation in pediatrics, a young patient of yours confides in you that they are feeling anxious and sad because they overheard their parents discussing financial problems at home. The child expresses worry about being a burden because of the medical bills.

Please rate the effectiveness of each response to this situation.

1. Reassure the child that their health is the top priority and that their parents want the best for them.
2. Tell the child that they shouldn't eavesdrop on their parents' conversations.
3. Discuss the child's feelings with the parents without the child's consent.
4. Connect the child with a counselor or social worker to discuss their feelings.
5. Avoid discussing the issue further and focus only on the medical treatment.

Answer Key & Explanations for Practice Question 30

Reassure the child that their health is the top priority and that their parents want the best for them.
Very Effective (4): Providing emotional support and reassurance is essential, especially for pediatric patients who may not fully grasp the complexities of adult problems.

Tell the child that they shouldn't eavesdrop on their parents' conversations.
Ineffective (2): While it's not ideal for children to overhear potentially distressing conversations, scolding the child doesn't address their immediate emotional needs.

Discuss the child's feelings with the parents without the child's consent.
Effective (3): Though it's crucial to involve parents in their child's care, one must approach this carefully to ensure the child doesn't feel betrayed or that their trust was broken.

Connect the child with a counselor or social worker to discuss their feelings.
Very Effective (4): Offering additional support resources, like counseling, can help the child process their feelings and concerns.

Avoid discussing the issue further and focus only on the medical treatment.

Ineffective (2): Ignoring the emotional needs of a patient, especially in pediatrics, may hinder the overall care and well-being of the patient.

Practice Question 31

You're a medical student shadowing a surgeon. During a consultation, the patient is visibly nervous about an upcoming surgery. The patient shares with the surgeon that they've read multiple horror stories online about surgeries gone wrong and is now having second thoughts about going through with the procedure.

Please rate the effectiveness of each response to this situation.

1. Dismiss the patient's concerns, stating that online stories are often exaggerated.
2. Offer the patient a list of credible sources where they can find accurate information about the surgery.
3. Share personal anecdotes about friends or family who had positive surgery outcomes.
4. Encourage the patient to express their fears and ask any questions they might have.
5. Suggest the patient postpone the surgery if they're feeling too anxious.

Answer Key & Explanations for Practice Question 31

Dismiss the patient's concerns, stating that online stories are often exaggerated.
Ineffective (2): Dismissing the patient's concerns outright may lead to a breakdown in trust and may not alleviate their fears.

Offer the patient a list of credible sources where they can find accurate information about the surgery.
Very Effective (4): Providing accurate and reliable information can help dispel myths and allow the patient to make an informed decision.

Share personal anecdotes about friends or family who had positive surgery outcomes.
Effective (3): While personal anecdotes can be comforting, they may not be as impactful as providing credible sources or clinical evidence.

Encourage the patient to express their fears and ask any questions they might have.
Very Effective (4): Open communication and understanding the patient's perspective can build trust and make them feel heard.

Suggest the patient postpone the surgery if they're feeling too anxious.
Effective (3): Although it's essential to consider the patient's emotional well-being, postponing surgery might not always be in the patient's best medical interest. It's crucial to balance emotional needs with medical needs.

Practice Question 32

You're in a study group preparing for an upcoming exam. One member, Alex, admits they're struggling with a particular topic and fears it might impact their grade. The rest of the group is comfortable with the material, and the exam is in two days.

Please rate the effectiveness of each response to this situation.

1. Advise Alex to seek out additional resources or tutoring since the group is moving ahead.
2. Allocate a small portion of the study session for everyone to help Alex understand.
3. Tell Alex they should've started studying earlier and that it's too late now.
4. Offer to meet Alex separately after the group session for a focused study.
5. Ignore Alex's concerns and continue with the planned study agenda.

Answer Key & Explanations for Practice Question 32

Advise Alex to seek out additional resources or tutoring since the group is moving ahead.
Effective (3): While suggesting additional resources is beneficial, it may come off as dismissive if not done empathetically.

Allocate a small portion of the study session for everyone to help Alex understand.
Very Effective (4): This approach fosters a collaborative learning environment and ensures no one is left behind.

Tell Alex they should've started studying earlier and that it's too late now.
Very Ineffective (1): This response is not supportive and can demotivate Alex further.

Offer to meet Alex separately after the group session for a focused study.
Very Effective (4): Offering individualized help shows empathy and commitment to your peers.

Ignore Alex's concerns and continue with the planned study agenda.
Ineffective (2): Ignoring a team member's concern can lead to a negative group dynamic and doesn't promote a supportive learning environment.

Practice Question 33

You are in the hospital's cafeteria and overhear two residents discussing a patient's condition openly, mentioning the patient's full name. They seem unaware that their conversation is violating patient confidentiality.

Please rate the effectiveness of each response to this situation.

1. Confront the residents immediately in the cafeteria and remind them of patient confidentiality.
2. Avoid getting involved and assume someone else will handle it.
3. Report the incident to your supervisor without talking to the residents.
4. Approach the residents privately after their meal and share your concerns about patient confidentiality.
5. Join their conversation, redirecting it to a safer topic without explicitly addressing the confidentiality breach.

Answer Key & Explanations for Practice Question 33

Confront the residents immediately in the cafeteria and remind them of patient confidentiality.
Effective (3): Addressing the issue promptly is essential, but doing so in a public setting may embarrass or escalate the situation.

Avoid getting involved and assume someone else will handle it.
Ineffective (2): Ignoring a breach of patient confidentiality is not responsible, and assuming someone else will handle it can perpetuate the issue.

Report the incident to your supervisor without talking to the residents.
Effective (3): Reporting is crucial, but addressing the residents directly might be a more immediate solution to ensure the behavior doesn't continue.

Approach the residents privately after their meal and share your concerns about patient confidentiality.
Very Effective (4): This approach is both proactive and respectful, addressing the issue without causing public embarrassment.

Join their conversation, redirecting it to a safer topic without explicitly addressing the confidentiality breach.

Effective (3): Redirecting is a subtle way to handle the situation, but it doesn't ensure the residents are aware of their error.

Practice Question 34

You are paired with a classmate for a month-long research project. A week into the project, you notice your partner frequently arriving late to meetings and missing deadlines, affecting the project's progress.

Please rate the effectiveness of each response to this situation.

1. Immediately report your classmate to the professor without discussing the matter with them.
2. Wait until the end of the month and mention their tardiness during the peer review process.
3. Approach your classmate and ask if they are facing any issues that are affecting their participation in the project.
4. Complete the majority of the project by yourself to ensure it gets done on time.
5. Send an email to your classmate detailing their missed deadlines and request they commit more time to the project.

Answer Key & Explanations for Practice Question 34

Immediately report your classmate to the professor without discussing the matter with them.
Ineffective (2): Jumping to reporting without first communicating with the classmate might escalate the situation unnecessarily.

Wait until the end of the month and mention their tardiness during the peer review process.
Ineffective (2): Waiting too long to address the issue can negatively impact the project's outcome and may not provide the classmate an opportunity to improve.

Approach your classmate and ask if they are facing any issues that are affecting their participation in the project.
Very Effective (4): Open communication allows for understanding and offers a chance for the classmate to share any challenges they might be facing.

Complete the majority of the project by yourself to ensure it gets done on time.
Effective (3): While this ensures the project's completion, it doesn't address the underlying issue and might result in an uneven distribution of work.

Send an email to your classmate detailing their missed deadlines and request they commit more time to the project.

Effective (3): Addressing the missed deadlines is necessary, but the tone and medium (email) can sometimes be misinterpreted.

Practice Question 35

During your clinical rotations, you are assigned to work with Dr. Thompson, a physician known for his strict demeanor and high expectations. You've heard stories from fellow students about how challenging it can be to meet his standards. You're eager to impress and learn but are nervous about the upcoming experience.

Please rate the effectiveness of each response to this situation.

1. Avoid asking Dr. Thompson any questions to minimize chances of making mistakes.
2. Proactively approach Dr. Thompson on the first day, expressing your eagerness to learn and asking for feedback throughout the rotation.
3. Focus only on the tasks where you feel most confident, avoiding anything new or challenging.
4. Share your concerns with fellow students, hoping to gain insights from their experiences with Dr. Thompson.
5. At the end of the first week, request feedback from Dr. Thompson on your performance and areas of improvement.

Answer Key & Explanations for Practice Question 35

Avoid asking Dr. Thompson any questions to minimize chances of making mistakes.
Ineffective (2): By not asking questions, you might miss out on crucial learning opportunities and risk making errors due to lack of clarification.

Proactively approach Dr. Thompson on the first day, expressing your eagerness to learn and asking for feedback throughout the rotation.
Very Effective (4): This approach shows initiative and willingness to learn, which can create a positive first impression.

Focus only on the tasks where you feel most confident, avoiding anything new or challenging.
Ineffective (2): Clinical rotations are an opportunity to learn and grow. By only sticking to familiar tasks, you miss out on valuable experiences.

Share your concerns with fellow students, hoping to gain insights from their experiences with Dr. Thompson.
Effective (3): While it's beneficial to gain insights from peers, relying solely on their experiences might not be the most constructive approach.

At the end of the first week, request feedback from Dr. Thompson on your performance and areas of improvement.
Very Effective (4): Regular feedback is essential for growth. This action shows that you value Dr. Thompson's opinion and are keen on improving.

Practice Question 36

You're part of a study group that meets twice a week. Lately, one member, Alex, has been frequently arriving late or missing sessions without prior notice. When present, Alex often seems unprepared and relies heavily on the group's notes and insights. Your study group is concerned about this pattern and its impact on the group's productivity.

Please rate the effectiveness of each response to this situation.

1. Discreetly ask other group members to exclude Alex from future meetings without discussing the issue directly with him.
2. At the beginning of the next session, set group ground rules regarding punctuality and preparation.
3. Send Alex a private message, expressing your concerns and asking if there are any personal issues affecting his attendance and preparation.
4. Address the issue publicly in the group, emphasizing that Alex's behavior is affecting the group's overall progress.
5. Offer to help Alex catch up outside of the group meetings, ensuring he is on par with everyone else.

Answer Key & Explanations for Practice Question 36

Discreetly ask other group members to exclude Alex from future meetings without discussing the issue directly with him.
Ineffective (2): Excluding a member without direct communication might lead to misunderstandings and harm group dynamics.

At the beginning of the next session, set group ground rules regarding punctuality and preparation.
Very Effective (4): Establishing ground rules can help set clear expectations for all group members, promoting productivity and cohesion.

Send Alex a private message, expressing your concerns and asking if there are any personal issues affecting his attendance and preparation.
Effective (3): Direct communication is essential. By reaching out privately, you show empathy and concern for Alex while addressing the issue.

Address the issue publicly in the group, emphasizing that Alex's behavior is affecting the group's overall progress.
Ineffective (2): Publicly addressing the issue might make Alex defensive and harm group cohesion. It's better to approach such issues in a more private manner.

Offer to help Alex catch up outside of the group meetings, ensuring he is on par with everyone else.

Effective (3): By offering help, you're demonstrating a cooperative and supportive attitude. However, it's essential to ensure that this doesn't detract from your study commitments.

Practice Question 37

While studying late in the library, you notice a fellow student who seems distraught. They are audibly muttering to themselves, seem frustrated, and occasionally wipe away tears. As you pack up to leave, you ponder whether you should approach them.

Please rate the effectiveness of each response to this situation.

1. Immediately inform the library staff about the student's behavior without approaching them.
2. Approach the student, introduce yourself, and ask if they're okay or if they'd like to talk.
3. Leave the library without intervening but mention the situation to a mutual friend.
4. Sit next to the student and start a conversation about your own stresses to create a mutual understanding.
5. On your way out, offer them a comforting gesture, like a reassuring smile, without directly addressing their distress.

Answer Key & Explanations for Practice Question 37

Immediately inform the library staff about the student's behavior without approaching them.
Ineffective (2): While the intention is to help, directly involving the library staff without understanding the context might escalate the situation unnecessarily.

Approach the student, introduce yourself, and ask if they're okay or if they'd like to talk.
Very Effective (4): Showing genuine concern and offering a listening ear can be comforting to someone in distress. It's a direct and empathetic approach.

Leave the library without intervening but mention the situation to a mutual friend.
Ineffective (2): While you might believe you're doing good by informing someone else, this may breach the student's privacy and not provide the immediate support they might need.

Sit next to the student and start a conversation about your own stresses to create a mutual understanding.
Effective (3): Sharing your own experiences might help them feel less isolated. However, it's essential to ensure the conversation remains focused on their well-being.

On your way out, offer them a comforting gesture, like a reassuring smile, without directly addressing their distress.

Effective (3): A simple gesture can sometimes make a big difference. It lets the student know that someone noticed and cared, even if words aren't exchanged.

Practice Question 38

You are part of a study group in medical school. During one of the sessions, a group member consistently interrupts others and dominates the conversation, not allowing for collaborative learning. The rest of the group seems visibly frustrated but nobody addresses the situation.

Please rate the effectiveness of each response to this situation.

1. Confront the dominating member publicly during the session about their behavior.
2. Quietly endure the session without bringing up the issue, hoping it resolves itself in the next meeting.
3. After the session, approach the member privately and express your concerns, suggesting ways they can contribute without overpowering others.
4. Suggest to the group that you all implement a "speaking stick" rule where only the person holding an item can speak, ensuring everyone gets a turn.
5. Send an anonymous note to the member highlighting the group's feelings.

Answer Key & Explanations for Practice Question 38

Confront the dominating member publicly during the session about their behavior.
Ineffective (2): While it's important to address disruptive behavior, doing so publicly can cause embarrassment and further tension in the group.

Quietly endure the session without bringing up the issue, hoping it resolves itself in the next meeting.
Ineffective (2): Ignoring the issue is likely to perpetuate the problem, continuing to hinder the group's productivity and collaborative spirit.

After the session, approach the member privately and express your concerns, suggesting ways they can contribute without overpowering others.
Very Effective (4): Addressing the issue privately shows respect for the individual's feelings while ensuring that the group's concerns are communicated.

Suggest to the group that you all implement a "speaking stick" rule where only the person holding an item can speak, ensuring everyone gets a turn.
Effective (3): This strategy provides a structured way for everyone to participate equally and can indirectly address the dominating behavior without singling out the individual.

Send an anonymous note to the member highlighting the group's feelings.
Ineffective (2): While this avoids direct confrontation, it doesn't allow for open dialogue and can lead to confusion or further tensions.

Practice Question 39

You are assisting with a research project in your medical school that involves collecting data from various patients. One day, while entering data, you notice a mistake you made earlier which might alter the results. Your professor has already complimented you on your accuracy and meticulousness with the project.

Please rate the effectiveness of each response to this situation.

1. Ignore the mistake and hope it doesn't have a major impact on the study's results.
2. Correct the mistake without informing anyone, hoping no one will notice.
3. Inform your professor about the error, apologize, and offer to correct it immediately.
4. Discuss the mistake with a fellow student to see if they think it's a significant error.
5. Delay the project timeline to review all the data entries you've made to ensure no further mistakes.

Answer Key & Explanations for Practice Question 39

Ignore the mistake and hope it doesn't have a major impact on the study's results.
Very Ineffective (1): Ignoring the mistake could have significant implications on the research, leading to misleading or inaccurate results.

Correct the mistake without informing anyone, hoping no one will notice.
Ineffective (2): While correcting the error is important, not informing those involved lacks transparency and can lead to mistrust or further errors down the line.

Inform your professor about the error, apologize, and offer to correct it immediately.
Very Effective (4): Taking responsibility for the mistake and being proactive about fixing it showcases professionalism, honesty, and integrity.

Discuss the mistake with a fellow student to see if they think it's a significant error.
Effective (3): Seeking a second opinion can provide clarity on the significance of the error, but it is still essential to inform the professor and take appropriate action.

Delay the project timeline to review all the data entries you've made to ensure no further mistakes.

Effective (3): Ensuring accuracy is crucial in research. While this might delay the project, it ensures the integrity of the study.

Practice Question 40

You are working on a team project with three of your classmates. During the initial brainstorming session, one classmate consistently dismisses your ideas without providing constructive feedback. You're starting to feel frustrated and undervalued.

Please rate the effectiveness of each response to this situation.

1. Publicly confront your classmate during the meeting, telling them that they are undermining your contributions.
2. Send a message to the group chat after the meeting expressing your dissatisfaction with the brainstorming session.
3. Privately approach the classmate after the meeting, discussing your feelings and seeking understanding.
4. Stop contributing ideas since they always seem to get dismissed.
5. Ask the group for feedback on your suggestions to understand if others share the same opinion.

Answer Key & Explanations for Practice Question 40

Publicly confront your classmate during the meeting, telling them that they are undermining your contributions.
Ineffective (2): While it's important to address concerns, confronting a team member publicly might escalate the situation and affect group dynamics negatively.

Send a message to the group chat after the meeting expressing your dissatisfaction with the brainstorming session.
Ineffective (2): While it's important to communicate feelings, airing grievances in a group chat may not address the specific problem and can create further tension.

Privately approach the classmate after the meeting, discussing your feelings and seeking understanding.
Very Effective (4): Addressing concerns privately and seeking mutual understanding can be a constructive approach, reducing chances of further conflicts.

Stop contributing ideas since they always seem to get dismissed.
Very Ineffective (1): Withdrawing from participation doesn't resolve the issue and can hinder the team's overall performance and your personal development.

Ask the group for feedback on your suggestions to understand if others share the same opinion.
Effective (3): This approach is diplomatic and provides insight into the group's perceptions. It can lead to improved communication and group dynamics.

Practice Question 41

You are a member of a study group preparing for an upcoming exam. As the date approaches, you realize that one group member is consistently absent from study sessions without giving any notice. The group is relying on each member to cover specific topics for review.

Please rate the effectiveness of each response to this situation.

1. Exclude the absent member from future study sessions without any discussion.
2. Divide the absent member's topics among the rest of the group without notifying them.
3. Reach out to the absent member to understand their reasons and see if there's any way to assist or adjust.
4. Publicly complain about the absent member in the group's chat, expressing disappointment.
5. Schedule a group meeting to discuss and revise responsibilities, ensuring that all topics are covered.

Answer Key & Explanations for Practice Question 41

Exclude the absent member from future study sessions without any discussion.
Ineffective (2): Excluding a member without understanding the reason for their absence may not be the best solution. Open communication is key.

Divide the absent member's topics among the rest of the group without notifying them.
Effective (3): While it ensures all topics are covered, it's better to communicate changes to responsibilities rather than making decisions unilaterally.

Reach out to the absent member to understand their reasons and see if there's any way to assist or adjust.
Very Effective (4): Direct communication and understanding can lead to constructive solutions and might address any unforeseen issues the member is facing.

Publicly complain about the absent member in the group's chat, expressing disappointment.
Very Ineffective (1): This approach can create tension and is not conducive to a positive group dynamic.

Schedule a group meeting to discuss and revise responsibilities, ensuring that all topics are covered.
Very Effective (4): Addressing the issue as a group and revising responsibilities ensures all topics are covered and everyone is on the same page.

Practice Question 42

While shadowing a doctor at a local hospital, you notice a nurse making potentially dangerous errors while administering medication to patients. You are unsure whether to bring this up, given your position as a student observer.

Please rate the effectiveness of each response to this situation.

1. Confront the nurse directly and express your concerns.
2. Silently note down the errors and continue with your observation.
3. Discuss your observations discreetly with the doctor you are shadowing.
4. Report the nurse to the hospital administration without talking to anyone else.
5. Discuss the situation with your school's clinical coordinator for guidance.

Answer Key & Explanations for Practice Question 42

Confront the nurse directly and express your concerns.
Ineffective (2): As a student observer, it might not be appropriate to confront a nurse directly, especially without understanding the full context.

Silently note down the errors and continue with your observation.
Ineffective (2): While noting down errors is a good first step, not taking further action may compromise patient safety.

Discuss your observations discreetly with the doctor you are shadowing.
Very Effective (4): The doctor is in a position of authority and can better evaluate the situation. This step ensures that the issue is brought to light without causing unnecessary conflict.

Report the nurse to the hospital administration without talking to anyone else.
Effective (3): Reporting the errors is important for patient safety, but doing so without discussing with someone familiar with the context might escalate the situation unnecessarily.

Discuss the situation with your school's clinical coordinator for guidance.
Very Effective (4): Seeking guidance from someone in your academic institution can provide direction on how to proceed while ensuring that patient safety and professional decorum are maintained.

Practice Question 43

You are part of a study group that meets regularly to review material for an upcoming exam. You've noticed that one member of the group, Alex, is consistently unprepared and often asks basic questions, slowing down the group's progress. Other members of the group have started to express their frustration privately.

Please rate the effectiveness of each response to this situation.

1. Ignore the issue, hoping it resolves on its own.
2. Publicly call out Alex during the next study session for being unprepared.
3. Speak to Alex privately, expressing the group's concerns and asking if there's a reason they're struggling.
4. Disband the study group without addressing the issue directly with Alex.
5. Suggest that the group sets specific topics for each session so members know what to prepare in advance.

Answer Key & Explanations for Practice Question 43

Ignore the issue, hoping it resolves on its own.
Ineffective (2): Avoiding the issue might lead to growing frustration among group members, affecting the group's dynamics and efficiency.

Publicly call out Alex during the next study session for being unprepared.
Very Ineffective (1): This approach could embarrass Alex and create a hostile environment, which isn't conducive to collaborative learning.

Speak to Alex privately, expressing the group's concerns and asking if there's a reason they're struggling.
Very Effective (4): Addressing the concern privately is respectful and offers Alex an opportunity to explain any challenges they might be facing. It can lead to a constructive solution.

Disband the study group without addressing the issue directly with Alex.
Ineffective (2): This doesn't address the root of the problem and penalizes all group members by ending the study sessions.

Suggest that the group sets specific topics for each session so members know what to prepare in advance.

Effective (3): This structured approach can ensure all members come prepared, potentially minimizing issues like the one with Alex.

Practice Question 44

You are shadowing a seasoned physician, Dr. Smith, as part of your medical training. During a consultation, you notice that Dr. Smith misses mentioning an important piece of information to a patient regarding potential side effects of a new medication. After the patient leaves, you're unsure if you should address this oversight with Dr. Smith.

Please rate the effectiveness of each response to this situation.

1. Immediately report Dr. Smith's oversight to the clinic's supervising authority without discussing it with him.
2. Casually mention to another colleague about Dr. Smith's mistake, hoping they'd address it.
3. Approach Dr. Smith privately, inquiring about the missed information and expressing your concern.
4. Do nothing and assume that Dr. Smith had his reasons for not mentioning the side effect.
5. Offer to speak to the patient yourself about the potential side effect.

Answer Key & Explanations for Practice Question 44

Immediately report Dr. Smith's oversight to the clinic's supervising authority without discussing it with him.

Ineffective (2): Reporting without understanding the entire context or discussing it with Dr. Smith might not be the best initial approach. It could unnecessarily escalate the situation.

Casually mention to another colleague about Dr. Smith's mistake, hoping they'd address it.

Very Ineffective (1): Sharing the concern with a third party instead of addressing it directly can lead to misinformation, gossip, or further misunderstandings.

Approach Dr. Smith privately, inquiring about the missed information and expressing your concern.

Very Effective (4): Engaging in a direct and respectful conversation with Dr. Smith ensures clarity and provides an opportunity for him to address the oversight, if it was unintentional.

Do nothing and assume that Dr. Smith had his reasons for not mentioning the side effect.

Ineffective (2): By not addressing the concern, there's a risk that the patient might not be adequately informed, which could lead to potential complications.

Offer to speak to the patient yourself about the potential side effect.
Effective (3): While this shows initiative, it's essential first to clarify the situation with Dr. Smith to ensure consistent communication.

Practice Question 45

During a group study session for an upcoming exam, one of your peers seems noticeably distracted. They mention feeling overwhelmed and stressed, particularly with their home situation affecting their studies. You want to offer support without overstepping boundaries.

Please rate the effectiveness of each response to this situation.

1. Tell the group about a time when you felt similarly overwhelmed to divert the attention from your peer's struggles.
2. Immediately suggest that your peer should seek counseling without further discussion.
3. Privately ask your peer if they'd like to discuss anything or if they need any resources.
4. Tell the group to focus solely on the upcoming exam and not discuss personal problems during study sessions.
5. Offer to help them catch up on any missed study materials or concepts they're finding challenging.

Answer Key & Explanations for Practice Question 45

Tell the group about a time when you felt similarly overwhelmed to divert the attention from your peer's struggles.
Ineffective (2): While sharing personal experiences can sometimes be helpful, this might come off as making the situation about yourself rather than addressing your peer's concerns.

Immediately suggest that your peer should seek counseling without further discussion.
Very Ineffective (1): While professional counseling can be beneficial, offering this as an immediate solution without understanding the full context might seem dismissive or presumptuous.

Privately ask your peer if they'd like to discuss anything or if they need any resources.
Very Effective (4): A private conversation shows genuine concern, offers support, and allows your peer to share without the pressure of the group setting.

Tell the group to focus solely on the upcoming exam and not discuss personal problems during study sessions.
Ineffective (2): While it's essential to stay focused during a study session, this response might come off as unsympathetic, potentially alienating your peer further.

Offer to help them catch up on any missed study materials or concepts they're finding challenging.

Effective (3): Demonstrating academic support can be a helpful way to alleviate some of the stress they're feeling, even if it doesn't address the root of their personal concerns.

Practice Question 46

You're in a group project, and one of the team members consistently arrives late to meetings and fails to deliver their part on time. The entire team's grade depends on the collective performance and timely submissions. You have observed that other team members are becoming frustrated.

Please rate the effectiveness of each response to this situation.

1. Confront the team member in front of everyone about their tardiness and lack of contribution.
2. Drop hints during meetings about the importance of punctuality and meeting deadlines without directly addressing the issue.
3. Privately discuss with the team member about their repeated tardiness and ask if there's any issue they're facing that's causing the delays.
4. Express your frustration on social media, tagging the team member in the post.
5. Organize a group meeting to discuss ways to improve team dynamics and collaboration, ensuring everyone gets a chance to voice their concerns.

Answer Key & Explanations for Practice Question 46

Confront the team member in front of everyone about their tardiness and lack of contribution.
Ineffective (2): While it's essential to address the issue, public confrontation may further alienate the team member and create more group tension.

Drop hints during meetings about the importance of punctuality and meeting deadlines without directly addressing the issue.
Very Ineffective (1): Indirect communication may not be effective, and the problematic team member might not recognize they are the cause of concern.

Privately discuss with the team member about their repeated tardiness and ask if there's any issue they're facing that's causing the delays.
Very Effective (4): A private discussion allows for open communication without public embarrassment. It's both solution-oriented and empathetic.

Express your frustration on social media, tagging the team member in the post.
Very Ineffective (1): Broadcasting issues on social media is unprofessional and can escalate the situation negatively.

Organize a group meeting to discuss ways to improve team dynamics and collaboration, ensuring everyone gets a chance to voice their concerns.

Effective (3): This approach addresses the issue at hand and promotes open dialogue among all team members, fostering better collaboration.

Practice Question 47

You're a medical student observing a surgery. During the procedure, the lead surgeon makes a comment that you believe to be inappropriate regarding a patient's physical appearance. Other staff in the room chuckle, but you find it uncomfortable.

Please rate the effectiveness of each response to this situation.

1. Laugh along with the rest of the team to fit in.
2. Speak up immediately and question the surgeon's professionalism in front of the entire surgical team.
3. Discuss your feelings privately with a mentor or trusted faculty member after the procedure.
4. Document the incident and report it through the proper channels without confronting anyone directly.
5. Stay silent and hope that such comments are not repeated in future surgeries.

Answer Key & Explanations for Practice Question 47

Laugh along with the rest of the team to fit in.
Ineffective (2): While this may temporarily ease any awkwardness, it doesn't address the underlying issue and indirectly endorses inappropriate behavior.

Speak up immediately and question the surgeon's professionalism in front of the entire surgical team.
Ineffective (2): Although it's essential to address inappropriate behavior, confronting the lead surgeon during an operation might not be the best approach and could potentially jeopardize patient safety.

Discuss your feelings privately with a mentor or trusted faculty member after the procedure.
Very Effective (4): Seeking guidance from a trusted individual allows you to express your concerns, obtain advice, and possibly find a solution without creating immediate conflict.

Document the incident and report it through the proper channels without confronting anyone directly.
Effective (3): Reporting the incident ensures that higher-ups are aware of the inappropriate behavior, promoting a safer and more professional environment.

Stay silent and hope that such comments are not repeated in future surgeries.

Very Ineffective (1): Ignoring the issue does not contribute to a professional environment or ensure that such behavior won't be repeated.

Practice Question 48

During a patient consultation, you notice the attending physician seems dismissive of a patient's complaints about chronic pain. The patient appears visibly distressed and mentions that previous doctors haven't taken their concerns seriously. You feel a strong empathy for the patient and believe their complaints should be addressed.

Please rate the effectiveness of each response to this situation.

1. Immediately interject during the consultation to support the patient's claims.
2. After the consultation, discuss your observations and concerns with the attending physician in private.
3. Recommend alternative treatments or physicians to the patient without the attending physician's knowledge.
4. Stay silent, assuming that the attending physician knows best due to their experience.
5. Engage in a follow-up with the patient to provide support and ensure they have the necessary resources.

Answer Key & Explanations for Practice Question 48

Immediately interject during the consultation to support the patient's claims.
Ineffective (2): While it's crucial to advocate for the patient, interrupting the attending physician during the consultation may create conflict and could be perceived as undermining the physician's authority.

After the consultation, discuss your observations and concerns with the attending physician in private.
Very Effective (4): Addressing your concerns privately with the physician allows for constructive dialogue and provides an opportunity to advocate for the patient without causing confrontation.

Recommend alternative treatments or physicians to the patient without the attending physician's knowledge.
Ineffective (2): While it's essential to advocate for the patient, recommending alternatives without the physician's knowledge can undermine the trust and teamwork in the healthcare setting.

Stay silent, assuming that the attending physician knows best due to their experience.
Very Ineffective (1): Not addressing the issue could perpetuate a potential oversight in patient care and fails to advocate for the patient's well-being.

Engage in a follow-up with the patient to provide support and ensure they have the necessary resources.

Effective (3): While it's critical to support patients, it's also essential to ensure alignment with the attending physician and the broader care team. Checking on the patient shows care but should be done in collaboration with the medical team.

Practice Question 49

You are a first-year medical student. During a study session, you overhear a group of third-year students discussing a recent exam and the specific questions that were on it. You will be taking the same exam in a few weeks. Listening to their discussion would give you an unfair advantage over your peers.

Please rate the effectiveness of each response to this situation.

1. Quietly listen to their conversation and take notes without them noticing.
2. Politely ask the third-year students not to discuss the exam around you as it compromises the integrity of the exam for you.
3. Immediately report the third-year students to the school administration for academic dishonesty.
4. Join the conversation and ask for more details about the questions.
5. Remove yourself from the environment without saying anything to avoid hearing the content.

Answer Key & Explanations for Practice Question 49

Quietly listen to their conversation and take notes without them noticing.
Very Ineffective (1): This is essentially cheating, as it provides an unfair advantage and is dishonest.

Politely ask the third-year students not to discuss the exam around you as it compromises the integrity of the exam for you.
Very Effective (4): Directly addressing the situation in a respectful manner is appropriate. It maintains the academic integrity of the exam and your personal ethics.

Immediately report the third-year students to the school administration for academic dishonesty.
Ineffective (2): While maintaining the academic integrity is important, directly reporting them without discussing the matter first might escalate the situation unnecessarily.

Join the conversation and ask for more details about the questions.
Very Ineffective (1): Actively seeking more information compounds the ethical issue. This is a clear violation of academic integrity.

Remove yourself from the environment without saying anything to avoid hearing the content.

Effective (3): By removing yourself, you're taking personal responsibility and ensuring you don't gain an unfair advantage. However, addressing the issue directly might be more beneficial for all involved.

Practice Question 50

You are assigned to work in a group for a major project. Two weeks into the assignment, you notice that one member, Alex, has not contributed to the group meetings or the project. Your final presentation is due in a week.

Please rate the effectiveness of each response to this situation.

1. Send an email to the professor explaining Alex's lack of contribution, requesting a grade penalty for him.
2. Confront Alex angrily in front of the entire group, expressing your frustration about his lack of contribution.
3. Arrange a private meeting with Alex to discuss his participation and find out if there are any issues or reasons for his absence.
4. Assign Alex the remaining tasks without his consent, ensuring he has a workload.
5. Discuss the situation with the rest of the group members and decide on a collective course of action.

Answer Key & Explanations for Practice Question 50

Send an email to the professor explaining Alex's lack of contribution, requesting a grade penalty for him.
Ineffective (2): Reporting without first trying to address the issue with Alex or the group might escalate the situation prematurely.

Confront Alex angrily in front of the entire group, expressing your frustration about his lack of contribution.
Very Ineffective (1): Confronting someone aggressively, especially in public, can be counterproductive and damage team dynamics.

Arrange a private meeting with Alex to discuss his participation and find out if there are any issues or reasons for his absence.
Very Effective (4): Addressing concerns privately and empathetically gives Alex a chance to explain and might lead to a productive resolution.

Assign Alex the remaining tasks without his consent, ensuring he has a workload.
Ineffective (2): Assigning tasks without discussion can lead to resentment and may not solve the core issue.

Discuss the situation with the rest of the group members and decide on a collective course of action.

Effective (3): Collaborative decision-making can be beneficial, but it's essential to ensure that the group doesn't gang up on Alex. It's also a good idea to discuss the situation with Alex after this.

Practice Question 51

You are in the middle of your clinical rotations and are assigned to work under Dr. Roberts. During rounds, Dr. Roberts frequently makes sarcastic remarks about patients' choices and seems dismissive of their concerns. Many patients have expressed discomfort with this behavior, but no one has formally reported it.

Please rate the effectiveness of each response to this situation.

1. Ignore Dr. Roberts' behavior and assume it's just his way of handling stress.
2. Engage in similar behavior, thinking it might be an accepted norm in this environment.
3. Speak privately with Dr. Roberts, expressing your observations and concerns about how the patients feel.
4. Share your observations with a trusted mentor or senior doctor and ask for advice on how to handle the situation.
5. Document each instance of Dr. Roberts' behavior, preparing for a potential formal complaint.

Answer Key & Explanations for Practice Question 51

Ignore Dr. Roberts' behavior and assume it's just his way of handling stress.
Ineffective (2): Ignoring the issue does not address the underlying problem or support patient welfare.

Engage in similar behavior, thinking it might be an accepted norm in this environment.
Very Ineffective (1): Emulating inappropriate behavior compromises patient trust and can have negative consequences for your own professional development.

Speak privately with Dr. Roberts, expressing your observations and concerns about how the patients feel.
Effective (3): Open dialogue can lead to understanding and change. However, approaching a senior doctor can be intimidating and may not always result in a positive outcome.

Share your observations with a trusted mentor or senior doctor and ask for advice on how to handle the situation.
Very Effective (4): Seeking guidance ensures you're not navigating the situation alone and can lead to a more informed approach.

Document each instance of Dr. Roberts' behavior, preparing for a potential formal complaint.
Effective (3): Documentation is essential if formal actions are needed later, but it's also important to address the issue directly when appropriate.

Practice Question 52

You are on a team working on a research project regarding a new drug's potential effects on heart disease. One of your team members, Alex, consistently misses deadlines and often provides incomplete data. Your research is time-sensitive, and these delays are affecting the project's progress.

Please rate the effectiveness of each response to this situation.

1. Discuss the issue with other team members behind Alex's back to see if they share your concerns.
2. Confront Alex in a team meeting, pointing out the mistakes and missed deadlines in front of everyone.
3. Arrange a one-on-one meeting with Alex to understand the reasons for the delays and offer assistance or solutions.
4. Send an email to the entire team, highlighting the importance of meeting deadlines without specifically naming Alex.
5. Approach your supervisor with your concerns about Alex's performance.

Answer Key & Explanations for Practice Question 52

Discuss the issue with other team members behind Alex's back to see if they share your concerns.
Ineffective (2): Discussing team issues behind a member's back can lead to gossip and erode trust within the team.

Confront Alex in a team meeting, pointing out the mistakes and missed deadlines in front of everyone.
Very Ineffective (1): Publicly confronting a team member can be embarrassing and may not address the root of the issue. It can also damage team dynamics.

Arrange a one-on-one meeting with Alex to understand the reasons for the delays and offer assistance or solutions.
Very Effective (4): Addressing the issue directly in a private setting is respectful and can lead to understanding and resolution.

Send an email to the entire team, highlighting the importance of meeting deadlines without specifically naming Alex.
Effective (3): Reminding everyone about the importance of deadlines can potentially benefit the entire team. However, indirect communication may not directly address Alex's specific issues.

Approach your supervisor with your concerns about Alex's performance.
Effective (3): If personal efforts to resolve the issue are ineffective, escalating concerns might be necessary. However, it's generally best to attempt to resolve interpersonal issues at the peer level before involving supervisors.

Practice Question 53

You are a medical student who has been assigned a group project with three other classmates. After several meetings, it becomes clear that one member, Jordan, does not seem to understand the core concepts of the assignment. The deadline is approaching, and you're concerned about how Jordan's contribution might impact the group's overall grade.

Please rate the effectiveness of each response to this situation.

1. Allocate more straightforward tasks to Jordan and don't involve them in the complex parts of the project.
2. Speak privately with Jordan to gauge their understanding and offer to help explain any confusing concepts.
3. Contact the professor and ask to be reassigned to a different group.
4. Suggest a group study session where everyone can review and discuss the assignment's main concepts.
5. Complete Jordan's portion of the project yourself to ensure it's done correctly.

Answer Key & Explanations for Practice Question 53

Allocate more straightforward tasks to Jordan and don't involve them in the complex parts of the project.
Effective (3): By giving Jordan tasks that match their current understanding, the project can still progress. However, this doesn't address the root issue of Jordan's lack of comprehension.

Speak privately with Jordan to gauge their understanding and offer to help explain any confusing concepts.
Very Effective (4): This approach is empathetic and proactive. It provides an opportunity to understand Jordan's perspective and directly address the issue.

Contact the professor and ask to be reassigned to a different group.
Very Ineffective (1): This avoids the problem rather than addressing it and can come off as not being a team player.

Suggest a group study session where everyone can review and discuss the assignment's main concepts.
Very Effective (4): This is an inclusive solution that can benefit all members of the group, reinforcing understanding and fostering collaboration.

Complete Jordan's portion of the project yourself to ensure it's done correctly.

Ineffective (2): While this ensures the work's quality, it doesn't allow Jordan to learn or contribute, and it may create an imbalance of work distribution.

Practice Question 54

As a medical student, you are rotating through various hospital departments. In the pediatrics department, you encounter a young patient who is very scared and refuses to be examined. The attending physician is getting impatient and wants to move on to the next patient.

Please rate the effectiveness of each response to this situation.

1. Ignore the child's fear and quickly perform the examination to keep up with the attending physician's pace.
2. Suggest a short break to allow the child to calm down before attempting the examination again.
3. Talk gently to the child, explaining the importance of the examination and assuring them that it won't hurt.
4. Ask the attending physician to handle the examination since they have more experience.
5. Bring in a toy or distraction to help soothe the child's fears during the examination.

Answer Key & Explanations for Practice Question 54

Ignore the child's fear and quickly perform the examination to keep up with the attending physician's pace.
Very Ineffective (1): This approach may further scare the child and make future examinations more challenging. It also lacks empathy and understanding.

Suggest a short break to allow the child to calm down before attempting the examination again.
Effective (3): This can help the child feel more at ease and might make the subsequent examination attempt more successful. However, it may not fully address the root cause of the child's fear.

Talk gently to the child, explaining the importance of the examination and assuring them that it won't hurt.
Very Effective (4): Establishing trust and explaining the process can help alleviate the child's fears. This approach is patient-centered and fosters understanding.

Ask the attending physician to handle the examination since they have more experience.
Ineffective (2): While the attending might have more experience, this doesn't guarantee the child will be more cooperative. It also avoids the opportunity for the student to learn from the situation.

Bring in a toy or distraction to help soothe the child's fears during the examination.

Very Effective (4): Distractions can be beneficial for pediatric patients, making the examination process smoother for both the child and the medical staff.

Practice Question 55

You're in a research lab, and you've been assigned to a team that's working on an important experiment. One day, you notice that a teammate has made an error in data recording, which can potentially impact the results. The data is about to be submitted for publication.

Please rate the effectiveness of each response to this situation.

1. Immediately correct the error without informing anyone to save time.
2. Speak with your teammate privately, pointing out the error and discussing how to address it.
3. Report the error to the principal investigator without discussing it with the teammate.
4. Bring it up during the next team meeting to collectively decide on the next steps.
5. Ignore the error, assuming that it might be a minor oversight and won't significantly affect the results.

Answer Key & Explanations for Practice Question 55

Immediately correct the error without informing anyone to save time.
Ineffective (2): While it's important to ensure data accuracy, making changes without discussing it with the team lacks transparency and can lead to trust issues.

Speak with your teammate privately, pointing out the error and discussing how to address it.
Very Effective (4): Addressing the issue directly with the person involved promotes open communication, allowing for clarification and collective decision-making.

Report the error to the principal investigator without discussing it with the teammate.
Ineffective (2): Going over the teammate's head without discussing the issue can create an environment of distrust and hinder team cohesion.

Bring it up during the next team meeting to collectively decide on the next steps.
Effective (3): This promotes transparency and collective problem-solving. However, waiting for a team meeting might delay addressing the issue, especially if the publication deadline is approaching.

Ignore the error, assuming that it might be a minor oversight and won't significantly affect the results.

Very Ineffective (1): Ignoring potential errors, especially in research, can lead to misinformation and discredit the study. Always prioritize accuracy and integrity in research.

Practice Question 56

You are a medical student participating in a clinical rotation. One day, while shadowing a senior physician, you witness them prescribe a medication to a patient in a dosage that you believe is incorrect based on your recent studies.

Please rate the effectiveness of each response to this situation.

1. Immediately confront the senior physician in front of the patient about the dosage error.
2. Silently make a note of it and later cross-check your information to ensure your understanding is correct.
3. Discuss your concern privately with the senior physician after the patient consultation.
4. Tell your peers about the potential error without discussing it with the senior physician.
5. Ask the senior physician during a private moment to explain the reasoning behind that particular dosage, indicating your desire to understand better.

Answer Key & Explanations for Practice Question 56

Immediately confront the senior physician in front of the patient about the dosage error.
Very Ineffective (1): Confronting a senior physician in front of a patient undermines the physician's credibility and can confuse or alarm the patient. It's essential to handle concerns privately and professionally.

Silently make a note of it and later cross-check your information to ensure your understanding is correct.
Effective (3): Double-checking your understanding is good practice. However, if there is a genuine error, it could go unaddressed, which may compromise patient safety.

Discuss your concern privately with the senior physician after the patient consultation.
Very Effective (4): Addressing the concern directly and privately with the senior physician is the most professional approach. It allows for clarification and ensures patient safety is prioritized.

Tell your peers about the potential error without discussing it with the senior physician.
Ineffective (2): Discussing the potential error with peers without first addressing it with the senior physician can lead to misinformation and damage the reputation of the physician.

Ask the senior physician during a private moment to explain the reasoning behind that particular dosage, indicating your desire to understand better.

Very Effective (4): This approach is non-confrontational and demonstrates a willingness to learn. It also gives the senior physician an opportunity to provide clarity or correct any oversight.

Practice Question 57

During a group study session, one of your peers becomes increasingly frustrated, claiming they can't grasp a particular concept. The upcoming exam is only two days away, and their anxiety levels are rising.

Please rate the effectiveness of each response to this situation.

1. Tell them that they probably won't understand it and should focus on other topics they're better at.
2. Take a short break, and then patiently explain the concept using different methods or examples.
3. Suggest they speak with the professor or teaching assistant for additional clarification.
4. Laugh it off and tell them it's an easy concept, and they're overthinking it.
5. Share your own experiences of struggling with challenging concepts and encourage them to persevere.

Answer Key & Explanations for Practice Question 57

Tell them that they probably won't understand it and should focus on other topics they're better at.
Ineffective (2): While redirecting focus can sometimes be a useful strategy, suggesting they "probably won't understand" is demotivating and can lower their confidence further.

Take a short break, and then patiently explain the concept using different methods or examples.
Very Effective (4): A break can provide a fresh perspective. Returning to explain the concept in various ways demonstrates patience and the desire to help, which can alleviate the peer's frustration.

Suggest they speak with the professor or teaching assistant for additional clarification.
Effective (3): Sometimes, getting an explanation from an authoritative figure or from someone who explains things differently can be helpful. However, it's essential to offer this suggestion sensitively.

Laugh it off and tell them it's an easy concept, and they're overthinking it.
Very Ineffective (1): This reaction dismisses the peer's feelings and can further decrease their confidence. It's crucial to be supportive and understanding.

Share your own experiences of struggling with challenging concepts and encourage them to persevere.

Very Effective (4): Relating through personal experiences can comfort and motivate them. Encouraging perseverance reinforces the belief that they can overcome challenges with time and effort.

Practice Question 58

You are in a clinical setting, shadowing a senior physician. The physician quickly diagnoses a patient based on their symptoms but doesn't explain the reasoning behind their diagnosis to you. You are curious and would like to understand the diagnostic process better.

Please rate the effectiveness of each response to this situation.

1. Decide not to ask since the physician probably knows best and might find your question bothersome.
2. After the consultation, respectfully ask the physician to explain the diagnostic process for your learning.
3. Interrupt the physician during the consultation to ask about the diagnosis.
4. Mention to the patient that you didn't understand the diagnosis, hoping the physician will explain.
5. Take notes on the symptoms presented and research them later on your own.

Answer Key & Explanations for Practice Question 58

Decide not to ask since the physician probably knows best and might find your question bothersome.
Ineffective (2): While it's essential to be respectful of the physician's time, not seeking clarity hinders your learning opportunity.

After the consultation, respectfully ask the physician to explain the diagnostic process for your learning.
Very Effective (4): Asking after the consultation is a polite way to ensure you don't interrupt patient care while maximizing your educational experience.

Interrupt the physician during the consultation to ask about the diagnosis.
Very Ineffective (1): Interrupting during the consultation is inappropriate and can disrupt the patient's care and the physician's process.

Mention to the patient that you didn't understand the diagnosis, hoping the physician will explain.
Ineffective (2): Discussing your uncertainty in front of the patient can undermine the physician's authority and the patient's confidence in the care they're receiving.

Take notes on the symptoms presented and research them later on your own.

Effective (3): Self-directed learning is a valuable skill in medicine. While this approach won't provide the immediate physician's perspective, it can be a useful supplement to understand the diagnostic process.

Practice Question 59

You are a medical student participating in a group study session. One of the group members, Alex, consistently dominates the discussion, not allowing others to share their perspectives or ask questions. You notice other group members becoming frustrated and disengaged.

Please rate the effectiveness of each response to this situation.

1. Confront Alex aggressively, telling them they talk too much and are ruining the group study.
2. Suggest to the group that everyone should have a designated time to speak to ensure diverse viewpoints are heard.
3. Complain about Alex to other group members behind their back.
4. Remain silent and decide to study on your own after the session.
5. Approach Alex privately, expressing your concerns and suggesting ways to ensure everyone gets a chance to participate.

Answer Key & Explanations for Practice Question 59

Confront Alex aggressively, telling them they talk too much and are ruining the group study.
Very Ineffective (1): Aggressive confrontations can create hostility and negatively impact group dynamics.

Suggest to the group that everyone should have a designated time to speak to ensure diverse viewpoints are heard.
Very Effective (4): This approach addresses the issue diplomatically, ensuring everyone has an equal opportunity to contribute without singling out Alex.

Complain about Alex to other group members behind their back.
Very Ineffective (1): Gossiping can breed resentment and further divide the group, exacerbating the issue.

Remain silent and decide to study on your own after the session.
Ineffective (2): While this avoids confrontation, it doesn't address the underlying problem, and you miss out on collaborative learning.

Approach Alex privately, expressing your concerns and suggesting ways to ensure everyone gets a chance to participate.

Effective (3): Direct communication can be helpful, but it's essential to approach the situation delicately to avoid making Alex defensive.

Practice Question 60

During your clinical rounds, you encounter a patient who is visibly upset. The patient tells you they received a new diagnosis that day, and they are struggling to process the information. They also mention feeling overwhelmed by the medical terminology and procedures the attending physician discussed.

Please rate the effectiveness of each response to this situation.

1. Tell the patient they shouldn't worry and that everything will be fine.
2. Offer to sit with the patient and explain the medical terms in a way they can understand.
3. Suggest the patient google their diagnosis to get a better understanding.
4. Express empathy and ask the patient if there are specific areas or terms they'd like clarification on.
5. Redirect the patient to speak with the attending physician without offering any immediate support.

Answer Key & Explanations for Practice Question 60

Tell the patient they shouldn't worry and that everything will be fine.
Ineffective (2): Although meant to reassure, this response can come across as dismissive and may not address the patient's feelings or concerns.

Offer to sit with the patient and explain the medical terms in a way they can understand.
Very Effective (4): Taking time to ensure a patient understands their medical situation can alleviate anxiety and promote trust.

Suggest the patient google their diagnosis to get a better understanding.
Very Ineffective (1): Recommending a patient to google medical information can lead to misunderstandings and additional anxiety due to unreliable sources.

Express empathy and ask the patient if there are specific areas or terms they'd like clarification on.
Effective (3): Expressing understanding and addressing specific concerns can help the patient feel heard and supported.

Redirect the patient to speak with the attending physician without offering any immediate support.

Ineffective (2): While it's sometimes appropriate to direct patients back to their primary physician for clarification, offering no immediate support can make the patient feel dismissed or isolated.